BERNADETTE MORGAN was trained in Hypnotherapy by Jonathan Royle PhD (creator of Complete Mind Therapy), Barrie St. John (creator of Hypno-Sensory Therapy), Andrew Newton (trainer of Paul McKenna), and Tom Silver (Trainer in Advanced and Scientific Hypnotherapy).

She is an advanced THETA HEALING™ practitioner teacher, an advanced practitioner in FREEWAY-CER©, as well as a practitioner in, EmoTrance and EFT (Emotional Freedom Techniques) and a member of the AMT (Association for Meridian Energy Therapies).

Healthy Mind, Beautiful Body

Healthy Mind, Beautiful Body

Bernadette Morgan

ATHENA PRESS
LONDON

WITH THANKS

Tom Bolton and Beverley Anderson for their kind permission to use the FREEWAY-CER© tapping routine within the text of this book.

Frank Lea, creator of Creative Mind Therapy, for his support, help, encouragement, and knowledge.

Bill Brookes for his wonderful work writing Bernie's song, and also, mixing the CD.

Special thanks to my father, my sons, and my wonderful partner Mícheál, for their patience while I obsessed over making this right.

Bernadette C Morgan DHP DCMT DHST APHP

INTRODUCTION

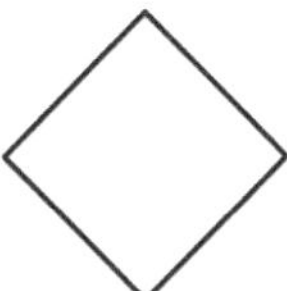

How many times have you said it to yourself? I wish I could lose weight! I feel ugly! I'm so fat! Well, I'm here to tell you that it is possible to change all of these things without pain or starvation. There is no reason to put yourself through agony to become a slimmer, happier person. It's all in your mind!

I know that sounds like a cliché, but it is the honest and absolute truth. You have the power to change anything you want to about yourself, however, before you can do that, you have to learn to love the person you are. With all the negative thought-patterns you have built up in your own mind, through years of being programmed by other people, is it any wonder that you, along with many of us, have a pretty poor self-image?

The aim of this book, and the accompanying CD is to change those thought-patterns. To, *reprogramme* your thoughts about yourself, your appearance, and your ability to succeed. You can be healthier, slimmer, more energetic, sexier, and more attractive just by imagining how you want to be. By embracing that image and allowing yourself to do what is needed to achieve it.

You may say to yourself, what does she know? Well, let me tell you. I am forty-four years old. I have children, a divorce, and a lot of other things going on in my life. I spent many years dieting, then gaining weight again because I failed to realise for all those years that my major problem was that I didn't like myself. I did not like *me*. I allowed the opinions and comments of others to devastate me and so I would hide inside myself and eat to make me feel better.

My mother died at an early age because she was obese. Her

body simply could not cope with the strain that it was being put under by the excess weight she was carrying. She suffered pain, ulcers and exhaustion constantly and was ultimately unable to care for herself properly. I have seen the harm that excess weight can cause, but more importantly I have seen the excess weight that poor self-image can cause. My mother spent as many years as I can remember going from one diet to another. She would lose four stone, even five or six at times, but it would always go piling back on.

The problem with diets is that they teach you to punish yourself for being who you are. By depriving yourself of the nutrition that your body needs and 'forbidding' you from eating things you enjoy. You count calories; allocate points to every single thing that passes through your lips. They take the control out of your hands and tell you that you must not eat this or that. They try to force you to eat what they have decided is good for you regardless of whether or not you actually enjoy. And so you sit there, feeling condemned, waiting to start this tortuous process that is going on a diet all over again.

Have you ever noticed when you are on a diet and have been told that you must not eat a particular food – even if you have not touched it for six months – you suddenly start to crave it? The moment you tell your conscious mind that this thing is 'forbidden', your unconscious mind says 'sod that!' and it will fill you with thoughts and desires that consume your every waking moment. It seems to be a fact of life that the moment we are told we cannot have something; we want it all the more. It's human nature!

The bottom line is that diets simply do not work long term. Sure, you will lose weight while you are starving your body, but what damage are you doing at the same time? There is a minimum level of nutrients that your body needs to maintain healthy function: 1500 calories, or worse 1000 calories a day is not going to provide that; and, more importantly your body will shut down in an attempt to protect its stores and keep you alive.

Diets may make you tired, depressed and bad tempered, and they will certainly cost you a lot of money if you attend classes. If that's not bad enough, when you stop you will most probably put all the weight you have lost, and more, back on.

What is needed is an approach that removes the pain from the process. A means of listening to the body and understanding what it needs so that you feel good about yourself. If you can achieve this, then the positive gains in self esteem will allow you to release those old patterns of eating and, with them, the weight you have been carrying around as protection from the world.

SO WHAT DO YOU THINK?

WOULD YOU LIKE TO JOIN ME ON THE JOURNEY?

We can do this together, you and I. It's a partnership from here on in. I will provide you with the tools you need to help you become the *BEST YOU* that it is possible to be. You are a wonderful creation, a beautiful person who deserves to be happy and healthy, and have all the energy and love that the world has to offer. You have to start right here, right now; for until you love yourself, how can you expect anyone else to love you?

Don't expect this to happen overnight – it won't. This is a gradual process of change in you, and in your life. There will be places along the pathway where you trip up and falter, but that's not important. What *is* important is your decision to make the changes you want. To be the person you know you can be.

Are you ready?

Great, then let's get moving, we have a long way to go!

SOME MYTHS DISPELLED

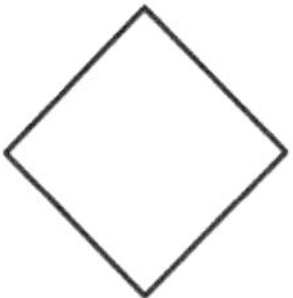

It is absolutely possible to eat whatever you want, whenever you want, and still lose weight, this sounds crazy but it's true.

The Healthy Mind, Beautiful Body system is so simple that you may find it hard to believe at first that it will work, possibly because you have been brainwashed into believing that weight loss is difficult. *IN REALITY IT IS NOT.*

Independent research into this system has proved it to be six to eight times more effective than dieting.

Some of the things you will learn may seem to conflict with things you have tried in the past or what you think is 'right'. You may have tried other methods of weight loss which failed to work or only worked temporarily before the weight came back.

Forget the things you have tried before. This is something dramatically different, surprisingly easy and most importantly, gives you permanent results. Changing not only your weight and how you think about yourself, but also giving you a whole new lifestyle and feel good factor.

SO LET'S GET STARTED

PREPARE YOURSELF FOR SOMETHING AMAZINGLY DIFFERENT

FORGET ABOUT DIETING – DIETS ARE SIMPLY TRAINING COURSES IN HOW TO GET FAT AND FEEL LIKE A FAILURE

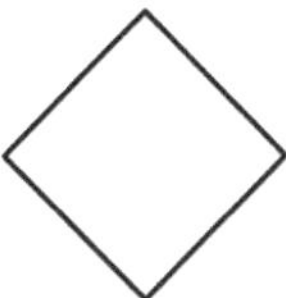

Any time someone tells me about a great new diet they have lost weight with, I ask them to tell me in six months time if they are still slimmer – so far not one of them has!

I believe there are far too many diets and too few results. There are thousands of diet books available, often with conflicting information. Is it any wonder people are confused and misguided? Even the multi-million pound weight-loss industry is confused and misguided.

Diets simply do not work long term, and many of them not even in the short term. Think of all those celebrities you see parading themselves in the media and on television, extolling the virtues of this product or that regime which has helped them win the battle with their weight. How frequently does it seem that all they've done is tried a diet, lost some weight, promoted that diet, and then put the weight back on. Then, they try another diet, lose weight, publicise that one, and then put the weight back on. And so on and so on. Meanwhile, they are getting paid huge amounts for endorsements, and the weight loss industry is earning millions; yet the only weight lost by the average person is the weight of the money missing from their bank accounts. Realistically most people cannot afford a personal trainer to put them through their paces, or a personal chef to prepare food which fits with this week's faddy diet.

SO WHY DON'T WE TRY A DIFFERENT APPROACH?

Whatever your aim – be it losing weight, becoming healthier, feeling really good about yourself, or maybe just trimming off those extra pounds – Healthy Mind, Beautiful Body can help you achieve it.

It is time to discover the truth about exercise and learn powerful techniques to help control cravings, resolve the emotional issues that cause you to comfort eat and supercharge your metabolism. Using these simple mind-programming techniques will reinforce the principles within this book and keep them working in your unconscious mind.

THE THREE THINGS MOST LIKELY TO PREVENT YOU FROM LOSING WEIGHT

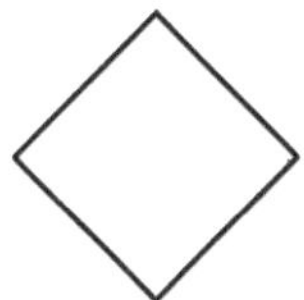

1. Obsessive Dieting

Most weight-loss books and systems seem to be filled with lists of forbidden foods, calorie counting guides and special menus. They so frequently say, 'This is not a diet'. Who are they kidding?

Regardless of what they may claim, any system which exerts control over what, when, or how much you eat is a diet.

Scientific research suggests that 90% of people who attempt to lose weight by dieting, fail.[1] The more times people fail with the many different diets they try the more they become convinced they will never be able to lose weight and the more despondent they get, maybe even thinking of themselves as failures or useless.

What we all need to understand is that the reason diet programmes do not work is nothing to do with you, as a person, it is to do with human biology.

During the Second World War, biological researcher, Dr Ancel Keyes PhD, found that people living on a semi-starvation diet became irritable, lost vitality and endurance, became obsessive about food, and even resorted to lying, stealing, and hoarding. A man who was a prisoner of war, forty years later, would steal food from the plates of other diners, hide his own food in his bedroom and eat everything he could, as fast as he could, despite the fact he was provided with three good meals every day.

---

[1] Schachter, S, Goldman, R, and Gordon, A, 'Effects of fear, food deprivation, and obesity on eating', *Journal of Personality and Social Psychology*, 1968.

Many other ex-prisoners of war reported that after release, when food was once more plentiful, they would eat up to eight times as much as they used to. An interesting fact is that the semi-starvation rations of the prisoners of war approximated 1500 calories a day which is MORE than some fashionable diets today allow.[2]

What does that tell us?

That simply depriving your body of food is the worst possible way to attempt to lose weight!

2. EMOTIONAL EATING

As a therapist, I have found that emotional eating is, probably, the biggest cause of obesity in people. Much of the time people eat because they are bored, unhappy, lonely, or tired. In most cases it has nothing to do with being hungry.

If a person eats because of an emotional need, the body will never feel satisfied by food – they don't get that 'full up' feeling to tell them to stop eating because the emotional need has not been satisfied.

An emotion is a need within a person that is crying out for attention and will continue to cry louder and louder until it gets what it needs. It will not go away until the *appropriate action* has been taken.

With this new understanding you will no longer have to be a victim of your emotions. From now on, when you feel the temptation to snack or eat a particular food, just stop and ask yourself: AM I REALLY HUNGRY? OR DO I JUST WANT TO CHANGE THE WAY I FEEL?

If you find that what you really want is to change the way you are feeling, no amount of food will do that for you.

Many of my clients have realised that their initial weight gain began as a result of a traumatic incident in the past, ranging from simple teasing or feeling that they were unwanted by their peers

---

[2] Keynes, A; Brozek, J; Henschel, A; Mickelsen, O; Taylor, H L, *The Biology of Human Starvation*, Minneapolis, University of Minnesota Press, 1950; also Schachter (above).

to serious trauma such as sexual, physical, or psychological abuse, and all areas between.

The mind-programming techniques in this book may help, but they are not a substitute for professional guidance. Therefore, if you suspect that something like this applies to you, please seek professional help from a relevant therapist.

3. FAULTY PROGRAMMING

Being overweight is not your fault. In many cases it will be the natural result of your emotional and mental programming and until that is modified, it is unlikely that external influences will change that. The only way to lose weight permanently is to access your unconscious mind and change your relationship with food for ever.

You are not a bad person. You are not useless, or a failure. You simply have some, currently, unhelpful habits. Fortunately, when you learn how to reprogramme your mind, you will be able to develop new, more productive ways of thinking and acting that will guarantee your success.

Simply follow what you learn in this book and you will simultaneously lose weight and any obsessions about food which you may currently have.

I will shortly explain the four most important things you need to know about losing weight and keeping it off for life. However, before I begin, let's take a few minutes to try out the following process.

THE POWER OF PERSPECTIVE

Imagine that it is many years from now, perhaps towards the end of your life, and you had decided *NOT* to bother with this system and begin to lose weight. Instead, you continued to try every diet plan that came along, continued to gain weight and lose your vitality and self-respect. As a result of that decision, how would you answer the following questions:

- What happened to your health?

- What were the consequences to your sense of well-being and self-respect?

- What effect did it have on your relationships?

- How does your body feel and function?

Now… just imagine that you learned and practiced this system, and easily reached and kept to your ideal weight:

- How good do you feel?

- What clothes are you able to wear?

- How much vitality and energy do you have?

- What are you able to do?

- What has your life been like having lived, all those years, at your ideal weight?

STOP!

Time to make a decision. Do you want to keep your excess weight and all the excuses for doing so? If so, you may as well not bother reading this book any further.

However, if you are ready to let go of all the excuses, get down to your ideal bodyweight, and enjoy the new life that goes with it, then you must realise that what you do from this point on is entirely in your hands.

Here we go…

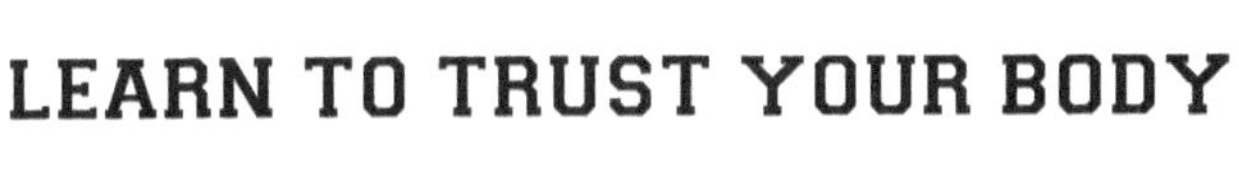
LEARN TO TRUST YOUR BODY

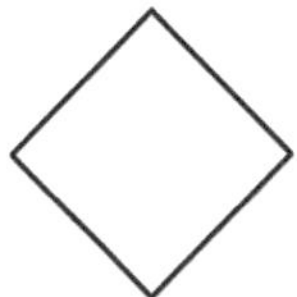

With so much conflicting information about 'wrong' foods and the effects on our health some foods are supposed to have, it can very difficult to understand or listen to what our bodies are telling us. Many of us are conditioned in to thinking that our bodies are bad or wrong, or don't fit the criteria laid down by fashion and the media. It can seem impossible to trust our bodies.

The truth is it's easy! Most new things seem difficult to start with. Learning to walk, tying your shoelaces, riding a bike... but once you practice it becomes easier, then second nature. Soon you are doing these things without even thinking about them.

The same applies to learning to listen to, and trust, your own body.

How do you get to eat like a naturally slim person?

Most naturally slim people rarely think about food apart from when they feel hungry. For them, making the right choices about food is a simple process. They seem to intuitively follow four basic principles which I will explain to you in the following chapter.

Make the force of habit work for you

When it comes to losing weight and keeping it off, habits can be your worst enemy. However, the techniques in this book will help you to reprogramme your habits so that they become your best friend and work for you.

I will be teaching you everything you need to do to easily change the way you eat, rather than what you eat, which will benefit you for the rest of your life.

All you need to do is follow the advice and guidelines I am giving you to easily make good choices about what and how much to eat at any time. You will quickly develop the habit of automatically eating in the right way for you.

Think of your stomach as a fuel tank. If you drove 100 miles a day in your car and it used 15 litres of fuel to do that 100 miles, but every day you put 20 litres of fuel in the tank, by the end of a year you would have put 1820 litres too much in the tank. How many extra tanks would the car need to hold that excess fuel? It is exactly the same with your body. If you put more food into your body than it needs, you will grow extra fuel tanks, and these will be situated in the stomach, hips, thighs and bottom. Does that sound at all familiar?

THE FOUR BASIC PRINCIPLES TO GETTING THE BODY YOU WANT AND KEEPING IT THAT WAY

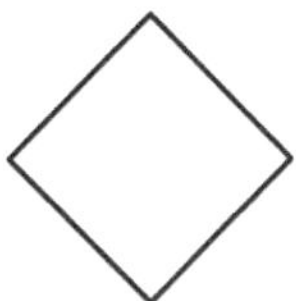

1. EAT THE FOODS YOU LIKE, NOT NECESSARILY THE FOODS YOU THINK YOU SHOULD EAT

In the 1930s, an experiment was carried out where a group of small children were given unlimited access to a huge range of foods from sweets, chocolate, jellies, cakes, through to cabbage, sprouts and beans. They were allowed to eat whatever took their fancy every day for one month.

At the end of the month, even though each child had chosen different foods at different times, they had actually eaten a perfectly balanced diet over the 30 days.[3]

You could also look to when a pregnant woman gets cravings for certain foods. No matter how strange these things may seem, it is simply the body telling her exactly what it needs to help the baby to develop.

It is pointless trying to resist!

When you decide you are not allowed to eat a certain food, the natural balance of the relationship with that food will be lost. Rather than wanting less of the 'banned' food, you will want more because human nature dictates that at least most of us, always want what we cannot have.

This produces an inner battle between your good intentions and your natural resistance to being controlled which can produce

---

[3] Elliott, Richard M, Goodenough, Florence L, Anderson, John E, 'Experimental Child Study' *The Century Co*, 1931.

all sorts of unpleasant and unhappy emotions.

As you learn to listen to your body and become comfortable about food you will become free of the guilt and tension that often results from not listening to your body and you will follow your intuition.

Once you are comfortable with following your natural inclinations about what and when to eat you will probably find your tastes changing. Like the children mentioned earlier, you will find yourself naturally eating a well balanced diet.

This is what some call the 90/10 balance where 90% of your food is nutritionally sound and 10% will be 'fun' or 'forbidden' food. In fact, you should not be surprised to find that you become naturally attracted to the very foods you are 'supposed' to be eating.

2. EAT WHEN YOU'RE HUNGRY – NOT OUT OF HABIT

Why do people eat when they are not really hungry? One of the main reasons people eat when they are not hungry is simply habit.

The habit of eating only at certain times of the day is for the most part, purely a case of convenience. We tend to eat when everyone gets in from work or school: lunch time is 12.30 to 1.30; break is at 11 o'clock, etc. From the body's point of view this is all faulty programming and tends to override the body's own natural function, desensitising people's ability to listen to and pay attention to their bodies.

If you think along the lines of, *I'm always hungry*, or *I'm never hungry* this could be what has happened to you.

As you begin to learn, again, how to listen to your body and be aware of what it is telling you, it will become easier to recognise the signals that indicate authentic hunger.

Depriving yourself of food (i.e. dieting) can actually make you gain weight.

When you deliberately go without food, you ignore the fact that you are hungry. If you do this for some length of time, your body begins to store fat for future energy needs. After a while your body will become stuck in this mode.

Your body appears to go into 'survival' mode – thinking the

supply of food is unreliable it stores fat 'just in case'. Over time it will begin to store more fat from the food you eat to add to the reserves.

Even when you eat so-called low-fat foods or reduced-fat ready-meals, if you are eating them at conventional mealtimes and not when you are hungry, your body will take all the fat it can to put in the store for later. This store, of course is the stomach if you are male, and the hips and thighs if you are female.

Part of the reason that slim people can eat a lot and not put on weight is because the body is not 'starving' and so has a choice about whether to store the fat for future use or eliminate it. Of course, if that person is very active, the body will take the fat it needs to provide the energy required, and dump the rest.

Overriding the body's natural call for food alters the metabolism. A fast metabolism burns more calories each day than a slow one, and by not eating when you are hungry you will cause the metabolism to slow down so that your body can conserve energy. This is why people often feel lethargic, producing symptoms of a mild depression.

Deliberately depriving yourself of food when you are hungry creates dysfunctional thought-patterns related to food in the unconscious mind. This unconscious tension related to food creates powerful chemical changes in the brain which lead to false hunger signals, cravings and bingeing. A vicious cycle develops: the less you listen to and trust your body, the more unreliable the body signals become, and so it continues.

However, all is not lost. There is a simple, easy way to break the cycle: simply eat whenever you feel genuinely hungry!

In a very short time you will feel more at ease, your metabolism will stabilise, and your body will take only what it needs to meet its current requirements and will then eliminate the rest.

3. STOP EATING WHEN YOU THINK YOU ARE FULL

As a therapist, I have seen many compulsive disorders. A huge proportion of those cases related to foul habits are due to faulty programming, often instilled during childhood. Many people have been conditioned to eat until everything on the plate is gone

– 'don't waste that food, there are starving children in the world,' 'eat it up or you wont get any pudding,' 'I didn't spend all day cooking for you to leave it on the plate.'

Remember that? I clearly remember being told that I would sit at the table until I had cleaned my plate. Three hours later my mother gave in because I simply sat there looking at it with a stubborn resolve not to eat what I didn't want. Some of this conditioning remains a powerful influence, even into adulthood.

The body is designed to eat when we are hungry and stop when we are satiated. This sort of faulty programming gets us out of touch with what our bodies really want and disrupts the entire system.

In order to lose weight, and keep it off, we must get back in touch with our body and work with it, not against it. To get that slimmer self, and keep it, we have to learn to listen again and be sensitive to our bodies, so that we can stop eating when we are full – being full is not the same as being stuffed, bloated, and can't get another mouthful in. This way we can eat only what we need to, and feel good and energised all day.

So how do we get to know what's going on with our bodies? Simple: when we have eaten enough the stomach sends a signal in the form of a gentle, satisfied feeling that lets us know the stomach is full.

If you miss this signal and continue eating you will find that each mouthful becomes less enjoyable and your eating slows down. The more you pay attention to that the more obvious it becomes.

When you continue to eat after the 'satisfied' signal, the stomach will start feeling more and more uncomfortable, heavy, and bloated. As soon as you notice these feelings you must stop eating no matter how nice the food is or how much or little is still on the plate.

If you are worried you might feel hungry again in a half hour or so, wait. You can always eat something then. However, it is vital to eat only what you actually want, not what you think you should. Eat consciously, savouring every mouthful, and as soon as you suspect that you are full – STOP!

Here is a simple, but powerful tool you can use to help you know precisely when to eat and when to stop eating.

HOW HUNGRY ARE YOU?

1 – Faint from lack of nourishment

2 – Starving

3 – Quite hungry

4 – Slightly hungry

5 – Not hungry at all

6 – Comfortably satisfied

7 – Full up

8 – Stuffed

9 – Bloated, overeaten

10 – So full, feel sick

Have a look at that scale and think about how your body feels right now. Getting used to tuning in to what your body is telling you – where do you feel you are on that scale right at this minute?

Of course everyone is different. But as a general guide it is best to eat when you are at 3 or 4 on the scale – fairly hungry but, before you become uncomfortably so.

If you leave eating until you get to levels 1 or 2, your body will go into starvation mode, and you could end up eating more than you actually need, causing the body to store the excess as fat.

It is best to stop eating at around levels 6 or 7, when you feel satisfied but not over full.

If you have done a lot of dieting in the past, you could well have lost touch with the signals from your body. You may be unable to tell when you were really stuffed or how to read the signals that tell you when you are really hungry. In that case, it is well worth practicing tuning in to your body every hour or so until you get used to noticing the difference between those points on the scale.

As you practice tuning in to your hunger messages, you will soon be able to recognise what your body is telling you long before you get to the desperately ravenous stage where your stomach grumbles and you perhaps feel a bit weak.

A very good practice is to eat small amounts of healthy food at regular intervals throughout the day, every 90 minutes to 2 hours. This will ensure that your blood sugar levels remain constant and your energy levels remain high. This prevents those peaks and troughs that happen when you eat a lot – and your blood sugar levels rise – or you don't eat when you need to – and your blood sugar levels crash and you feel tired or low.

By keeping your energy levels constant you will avoid that *got to eat now* feeling where you are tempted to grab the first thing, usually chocolate or similar, which gives you that quick boost, but is inevitably followed by a low. In short, you will avoid throwing your body out of sync.

I know many people who are what you might call naturally thin. These people generally eat small amounts quite regularly throughout the day, almost like snacking. They seem unable to eat really large meals, even on special occasions. They do eat a substantial amount throughout the day, but it seems that because they mostly eat small, frequent meals their stomachs do not expand very much. As such, they soon feel stuffed and overfull when eating large amounts. They also drink plenty of water during the day (remember the average person needs at least two litres daily).

These people are always fit, healthy, and have abundant energy, supporting my advice that eating small amounts regularly throughout the day is the right way forward.

Here's is another piece of advice: when you go shopping for food, do it when you are not hungry! That way you will not be so tempted to buy foods which you do not really need, especially unhealthy snack items. It also helps if you are not over-hungry when you visit a restaurant, or the local take-away, for the very same reason. You will end up ordering just the right amount to satisfy your system. A small point, but valid none the less.

4. CONCENTRATE ON YOUR EATING – ENJOY EVERY MORSEL

Some overweight people seem to spend a great deal of time thinking about food, and yet, when they are actually eating, they do not seem to think about what they are doing at all. It is as if they go into some sort of trance where they eat as much as they can get without chewing or tasting what is in their mouths.

The main reason for this is that whenever we do anything that we need to do for survival – eating, breathing, sex – a 'happy' chemical called *serotonin* is released in the brain. Overweight people tend to eat more in order to get a *serotonin high*. However, because of this high, they either do not notice or choose to ignore the signals from the stomach that say, 'Stop, I'm full.' This leads to them eating far more than they need, which causes the stomach to expand and the body to keep gaining weight.

Unfortunately the *serotonin high* is only temporary. The after effect leaves them feeling fat and guilty. Sometimes it is this after effect that leads to a repeat of the whole process, a vicious cycle of comfort eating in order to remove the bad feelings and bad feelings over the comfort eating.

The major advantage of the Healthy Mind, Beautiful Body system is that you can eat whatever you want, just so long as you take it slowly and enjoy every single mouthful.

This is important – you must really enjoy and savour the taste, texture and wonderful sensations of every mouthful by slowly, thoughtfully, and thoroughly chewing every morsel. You have to *notice* what you are eating to be able to really enjoy your food.

A study in Sweden, showed that blindfolded people ate approximately 22% less food than when they could see what they were eating, proving that when the test subjects had to concentrate on the taste and texture of their food they actually ate less.[4]

As you practice eating slowly, and carefully chew your food, you begin to consciously enjoy it. You will notice how good your food tastes and, most importantly, you will easily notice when you are full and stop eating.

Practice this:

For the next week or two, eat much more slowly than you usually do and thoroughly chew and taste every mouthful.

Deliberately put your knife and fork down between each mouthful (or put your sandwich back on the plate). Give yourself

---

[4] Linné, Y, Bakeling, B, Rössner, S, Rooth, P, 'Vision and Eating Behaviours', *Obesity Research*, vol. 10 no. 2 (2001), pp.92–95.

time to notice what you are doing. Only when your mouth is completely empty, should you put some more food in it. By doing this you will be making a conscious choice about whether to eat any more or not, instead of just thoughtlessly eating.

It is very important that you carefully chew your food.

Imagine you are watching TV and eating crisps or sweets, when the programme or film is over you suddenly realise just how much you have eaten without actually noticing you were doing so. When you are consciously aware of every mouthful it becomes almost impossible to binge eat, resulting in great benefit to your health and well-being. Try not to eat in front of the television, but instead eat at the table and pay attention to the process.

In addition, thoroughly chewed food is broken down more easily, which means your digestion will improve, and the body will be able to extract more nutrients from the food, which will in turn improve your energy levels. You will actually eat less and feel better altogether.

CHANGING UNWANTED EATING HABITS

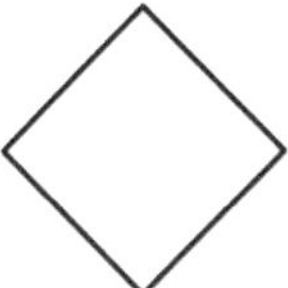

I have seen many serial dieters who, despite their constant dieting, still lost the battle with their weight over time. Some of these people, even by just following the four steps listed earlier, soon begin to lose their excess weight and find that they just don't want to overeat any more!

Many people suffer from what I call 'guilt eating' whereby they have to finish everything on their plates whether they are full or not. In many cases this comes from childhood where the child is told to eat everything and waste nothing because there are children starving in the world. This sort of thing becomes instilled in young people and they become stuck with that habit throughout life. It never occurs to them how being overweight can possibly help starving children in other parts of the world.

There has never been any evidence to suggest that eating everything on your plate has in any way helped people who may be starving elsewhere.

Surely the best thing to do would be to learn to manage your eating so that you eat only when you are hungry, enjoy every mouthful and stop when you are comfortably full. That way you won't eat so much, then, there will be more food to go round.

The easiest way to break the 'guilt eating' habit is to deliberately leave a small amount of food on your plate after every meal, this will tell your unconscious mind that you are changing and no longer feeling guilty about leaving some food on the plate.

Very soon the 'guilt' habit will be broken and you will be able to eat only what you need, putting less food in your stomach; and taking more control over your life.

Let's face it, once the food has been prepared it is already effectively 'wasted' whether you eat it or not because almost as soon as it reaches the table it is becoming stale and old. Therefore you are not making things worse by leaving some on your plate but you are making yourself fitter, happier and more in control.

MORE HELPFUL INFORMATION

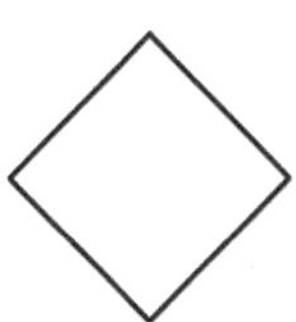

The human body is made up of about 75% water and, more importantly, the brain is almost 85% water. This means that when the brain senses an impending water shortage, it will begin to ration the water already in the body, giving priority to itself and directing just enough to the other organs to keep them functioning. Because of this, many of the minor aches and pains, including hangover pangs that we experience practically every day are actually the first symptoms of dehydration. This is why, sometimes, no matter what you eat it still does not feel quite right.

It is almost impossible to tell the difference between feeling thirsty and feeling hungry as the signals from the body are just about the same. Keep this in mind when you next get that feeling of hunger. It is a good idea to drink some fresh water, this will often remove the body's feelings of hunger telling you it was actually thirst. If you still feel hungry after drinking then it is hunger, so go ahead and eat!

WHAT HAPPENS NOW?

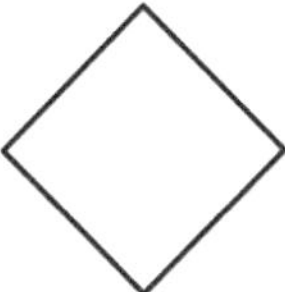

It could feel a bit strange to begin with.

The very best way to eat, is to eat slowly, chewing and savouring every mouthful, even to the extent of putting your knife and fork down between bites. Some people feel a bit self-conscious eating this way, perhaps feeling that people are staring at them.

To be honest, if you knew how little other people think about anyone else you would not worry about what they are thinking of you. Most people are so wrapped up in their own little worlds that they don't even notice what they are eating, let alone notice what you are doing. I often think to myself when in a crowd that to each person in this crowd the rest of us are invisible, and most of the time this is true.

In addition, friends and family who know you as a dieter and see you eating chocolate, pizza and cream cakes will probably think that you have failed on yet another diet. This time, however, you have the last laugh. As you practice eating consciously, slowly chewing and enjoying every morsel, you will find that not only does your food taste better, but you enjoy it more and experience the wonderful satisfying feeling that comes with being completely in control of your relationship with food.

That, of course, does not mean that you can continue to eat only 'rubbish' and lose weight. Let's be sensible here. You are learning to listen to what your body *needs*, and the 'junk food' that you have become addicted to is not it.

Today in our society we get constant messages about eating and body image thrown at us. What is often considered *normal* is actually nowhere near what is, in fact, *natural*. It may well feel strange at first to eat in this more intuitive way, but it is very important to realise that you are actually eating in a more natural and healthy way.

That is why I call this method, 'Healthy Mind, Beautiful Body'. Unlike diets, which tend to lead you away from eating when you're hungry and stopping when you're full, this method is one that you will easily be able to sustain throughout your life, without filling your mind with guilt and distress – it is possibly the simplest, most effective weight-loss method you will ever find.

You *WILL* feel better and better.

A consistent benefit of following this simple and effective weight-loss system is that your body will feel better as you progress and you will also feel better and happier about yourself with your self-esteem growing in leaps and bounds giving you a Healthy Mind!

- For probably the first time in years you will begin to feel more in control around food.

- You will rapidly see that it really is possible and easy to lose unwanted weight.

- You will stop worrying about what to eat and when.

- You will be free of the pressures and obsessions about food.

- You will realise that you are no different from slim people. You have the same ability as everyone else to lose weight.

- You will be totally amazed at how easy it really is.

Not wasting so much energy worrying about food, will leave you with more energy to get on with and enjoy your life. That extra energy will also be a good sign that what you are doing is working effectively for you.

You might wonder how successfully this system is working for you.

Do not be put out if you find that for the first week or two you are not entirely sure that it is working. It is natural to have doubts when you are doing something different. You might feel that you are eating more, or that you are not eating a nutritionally sound diet. You may even feel like nothing much is happening to your body or your mind.

But if you keep it up, it won't be long before you notice that you have more energy, your clothes begin to feel looser, and you are already beginning to feel better in your body. You will soon realise that the system is working.

Even though you may have tried all sorts of diets and regimes that have failed, by committing yourself to following the Four Basic Principles over the next two or three weeks, you will have nothing to lose except your excess weight.

Sometimes you might forget to follow the guidance in this book and break one of the Four Basic Principles.

Be prepared to accept that you will slip up now and again and find yourself eating the odd chocolate bar you didn't need, eating on the run, or even indulging in a full-scale binge.

You will then have a choice to make!

Either you can curse yourself, call yourself all sorts of names idiots, and convince yourself that you are never going to succeed. Or you can have a laugh, remember I told you this could happen, go back to following the Four Basic Principles, and get on with getting that Beautiful Body!

REMEMBER

YOU CAN ONLY FAIL IF YOU STOP TRYING!

NOW, ABOUT THOSE SCALES

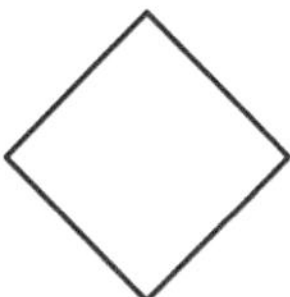

Many diets and weight-loss schemes seem to put a great deal of emphasis on weighing yourself. Some people even become obsessed with weighing themselves every day or after every meal, hoping to see that they have suddenly lost several pounds. Weighing yourself every day will not give you an accurate assessment of how you are doing.

Everybody's weigh fluctuates a little, all the time, even slim people. It is interesting to note here that most naturally slim people do not have a clue about how much they weigh; they don't bother with scales.

If you keep weighing yourself every five minutes you will only be setting yourself up to feel bad about yourself, disheartened and disillusioned.

All sorts of things affect your weight on a daily basis: fluid retention, the environment, even atmospheric pressure. Weighing yourself is the most unreliable way to check on the effectiveness of your weight-loss efforts. Apart from anything else if you are doing exercise and building muscle you will discover that you look better and trimmer but may not weigh any less. Here's a newsflash for you: muscle is heavier than fat! (As muscle is denser than fat, it takes up less space per kilo than fat would in the same area).

SO DO NOT WEIGH YOURSELF FOR THE NEXT WEEK OR TWO

In fact, I would go so far as to suggest you throw your scales away – the only truly accurate way to measure your progress is in the way you look and feel – when you can see you look slimmer, your clothes are getting loose, other people comment on how good you look, and most importantly, you feel good in yourself.

It is only natural that some days you will feel much better about yourself and your progress than others. And that is OK. If you stick to the rules and suggestions in the Healthy Mind, Beautiful Body method, you cannot help but lose weight and keep it off. Furthermore, as you use this system it will soon become a natural part of your life and you won't even have to think about it. The whole thing will become as natural as breathing.

IS IT REALLY THAT EASY?

OK, to quickly recap:

1. Eat whenever you are hungry.
2. Eat only what you want, not what you think you want.
3. Eat slowly, chew thoroughly and savour every morsel.
4. Stop the moment you think you have eaten enough.

Think of it as monitoring your body's fuel tank – when it's empty, add some fuel. That way you will only put in as much fuel as your body uses without storing any excess.

That's it, really. If you truly want to lose weight and stay slim for the rest of your life this is all you need to do. If you choose to do only one of the above, make sure it's number three.

By eating consciously and carefully everything else will natu-rally follow simply because:

- You can not get the same enjoyment from your food unless you are actually hungry.

- You can only enjoy your food if you eat the foods that you actually like.

- Your food will no longer be enjoyable once you are full.

PROGRAMMING YOUR
UNCONSCIOUS MIND TO HELP YOU
GET SLIMMER

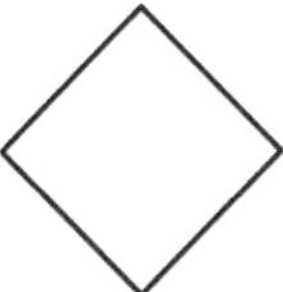

In the following pages I will share with you some of the amazing techniques that will help you programme your mind to ensure you become healthier and slimmer.

Your unconscious mind is the most powerful friend you have and by learning how to access it and letting it know what you want it to do for you, you are able to harness that virtually unlimited power to achieve whatever you want.

Let's begin by changing any unhelpful habits you may have picked up from dieting.

There are likely to have been times in the past when you have done your best to get yourself out of 'bad' eating habits, to lose weight by dieting or eating 'properly', and found yourself unable to stick to it. All these times you will have probably thought that it was somehow your fault, that if only you had more willpower you would be able to do it.

NOT TRUE!

It is actually almost impossible to break any kind of habit by willpower alone. You need to reprogramme your mind to remove the unwanted habit and replace it with the desired one. Think of your mind like a computer, if the right programme is running it is easy for it to do the right thing, with the wrong one running there is not much chance.

Life-long habits such as smoking, fears, and phobias have been changed, sometimes in only a few minutes by effectively repro-gramming the unconscious mind. Yet unless you experience it for yourself, it may seem hard to believe or understand. You may think that if changes can be brought about so easily and quickly then why have you not been able to do so before.

The simple answer is that your imagination is far stronger than your willpower.

Try this and see:

Imagine you have a bar of chocolate (or some food you absolutely love) in your hand, now call up all your will-power to resist eating that chocolate. Now imagine how good that chocolate will taste, savour the tempting smell of it. Imagine how wonderful it will be to feel it melting in your mouth, the lovely flavours and texture as you joyfully chew it. Having difficulty not wanting to eat that chocolate?

Now imagine again that you have that chocolate, but it is now covered in a smelly grey mould and covered in unpleasant-looking bugs. Do you feel any temptation to eat it? Probably not.

That is the power of your imagination; in fact, it is your imagination that helps you decide what to eat when you are reading a menu. As you read the menu your imagination gives you a taste of what the different food items will taste like and the one that appeals most will, of course, be the one you choose. That is why restaurants describe their offerings in the most tempting terms they can, for instance, which would you rather have? A succulent steak in red wine with garlic sautéed button mushrooms, or a cooked chunk from a cow's backside and fungus?

FOCUS ON WHAT YOU ACTUALLY WANT, NOT WHAT YOU DON'T WANT

In order to understand the above examples your mind has to focus on the very things you said you don't want. So when you think about the fat you want to get rid of, your mind is actually focusing on and strengthening the image you have of yourself being fat. This in turn can make you feel useless, ugly or unmotivated.

By the same token, when you focus on what you actually want – a slimmer, trimmer figure, being healthy and more active – your unconscious mind receives the image of you being slim, fit and healthy and will then do everything in its power to make that image a reality. So by creating a vivid and real image of yourself being exactly the person you want to be you are training your mind to develop and run a programme that will ensure that is what you achieve.

The more specific you are in your imagination and thoughts, the more effective this process is. So, for instance, by only thinking 'I want to lose weight' your unconscious mind does not know how much weight you want to lose or by when you want to lose it.

Therefore it is important to say exactly what you want: 'I want to lose two stone (28 pounds) in two months' or 'I want to be able to wear size (whatever) clothes' or even to be very brave and say, 'I want to love how I look when I'm naked.'

YOUR SELF-IMAGE

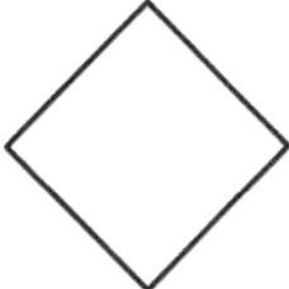

First a reminder of the Four Basic Principles:

1. Eat only when you are hungry.
2. Eat the foods you actually like.
3. Chew thoroughly and enjoy every mouthful.
4. Stop eating the moment you feel full.

By following those rules alone you will become slimmer and stay that way permanently, but by using the following techniques you will also make the whole process much easier, more effective and you will feel even better about yourself.

Why? You have probably heard the saying, 'You are what you eat,' but it is equally true to say 'You are what you think.'

Maxwell Maltz, a famous plastic surgeon, noticed that after surgery the patients were hugely more self-confident. A few however, still did not feel good about themselves. After studying those patients, Dr Maltz realised that those people had a *very poor self-image* and the fact that their appearance had been improved seemed to make little difference. It was apparent that those people needed help with what was wrong on the *inside* as well as the outside.[5]

Your self-image is the way you perceive yourself. It is what determines everything that you are – confident, motivated, happy or even lucky.

---

[5] Maltz, M, *New Faces, New Futures; rebuilding character with plastic surgery* New York, R.R. Smith, 1936

If you perceive yourself as being ugly, useless, worthless, unhappy or unattractive, then you behave as though that were true thereby reinforcing those negative self-images and allowing the cycle to repeat.

There are millions of people who perhaps are not necessarily all that special on the outside, but because they think of themselves as being confident, attractive, and worthwhile they actually are attractive to others. People like being around them and respond to them in a positive way. This in turn reinforces their own self-confidence and that happy cycle keeps repeating itself over and over.

Whichever self-image you have, it keeps proving itself right by causing you to behave in a way consistent with that image.

Most overweight people believe that they will always be fat or unattractive and so destroy any chance they may have of changing that situation.

As soon as you get into the habit of focusing on what you do want – being slim, attractive healthy, confident and happy – then that is what you will become and you will have to get used to thinking of yourself in that way. You have to admit that sounds good.

USING YOUR POWERS OF VISUALISATION

Visualisation techniques have been proven to dramatically boost your ability to lose weight. When you vividly imagine yourself as being slim, attractive and so on, your brain gets a clear message that WILL affect your motivation, metabolism, energy levels, etc. This in turn causes physical sensations that affect your emotions and generates positive thoughts about yourself, reinforcing the programming which you are giving to your brain. This creates a wonderful cycle, which keeps reinforcing itself as you see the positive results. As you go on, the whole thing gets more powerful and more effective.

THE MAGIC MIRROR

The following is a simple exercise in visualisation that will programme your unconscious mind to begin the process of losing weight and keeping it off.

Read through the steps first so you are sure you know what to do then sit or lie down quietly and go through the visualisation process.

Close your eyes and imagine that you are looking at your reflection in a magic mirror.

The reflection you see is of you at your ideal weight and shape.

Notice how good you look, the clothes you are wearing, the confidence in your stance and posture.

When you are completely happy with the image you see in the mirror, step into the image in the mirror. Put that person on like a new outfit; see through the eyes of that person; hear through the ears of that person. Experience how good it feels to be your ideal weight and shape; experience the feelings of confidence, pride and joy of having the weight and figure you always wanted.

Make the colours brighter, hear the compliments of other people, feel how good it is to go about your daily life with so much energy, pride and confidence in yourself. Feel how wonderful it is to be that wonderful, vivacious, happy, confident, and attractive you.

When you create this vivid, 'almost real' image of yourself and experience the good feelings in your mind as if it is actually happening you are sending powerful messages to your unconscious mind that this is in fact the person you are. Your unconscious mind will automatically reprogramme itself to ensure that you become that person in the shortest possible time.

Do the above exercise every night before you go to sleep and every morning before you get out of bed. Repetition is the key to success. The more you do this, the more established a neural pathway in your brain becomes, reinforcing your vision. The brain creates new neurons and pathways through learned experience, this is way babies' brains' develop and grow so quickly as each new thing they learn creates a new neural pathway and so teaches them something new by repetition.

As you keep visualising yourself as being slim, fit and healthy, signals are sent to your unconscious mind, which will cause it to make you eat, feel and behave like that person you visualise yourself to be. As you begin to lose weight and feel better in yourself you will further reinforce the good effects as the new programme becomes more and more powerful.

Keep focusing on your target in this way. As you continue to follow the Four Basic Principles described previously you will soon notice how quickly you are moving towards your ideal weight.

EMOTIONAL EATING

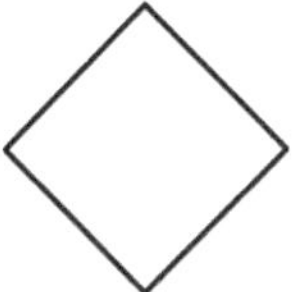

HOW TO RECOGNISE EMOTIONAL HUNGER

Emotional eating, as mentioned earlier, is one of the major causes of obesity, yet the diet books just keep telling you what you should not eat. They might as well try to fix the dent in the car by saying you shouldn't have been driving in the first place – what a load of nonsense! Instead of being over concerned about what you are eating, think about what may be eating you.

Physical hunger and emotional hunger can easily be confused, but as you become more attuned to your body you will soon begin to see the difference. One of the more easily recognised differences is that emotional hunger is urgent or instant whereas physical hunger is more gradual.

When you suddenly feel the need to eat or have a sudden urge for a certain kind of food, stop and think back a bit. Have you just been upset? Has something just gone wrong? Has the boss had a go at you or have you had words with your partner? Very often people try to bury these unhappy feelings by eating. This is emotional, or comfort, eating.

Physical hunger creeps up on you gradually, a bit of a tummy rumble or even a growl that gets more persistent the longer you ignore it. You may even get a bit tired, or start to lose concentration. As you learn to recognise these messages it will become easier to spot the difference between the two types of hunger.

You cannot satisfy emotional hunger by eating. If you find yourself continually eating and never feeling satisfied, it is because you don't actually need food – you need to change the way you are feeling. When you are suffering from bad feelings no amount of food will change them. In fact, too much food could make you feel even worse. Unlike physical hunger, which comes back as you use up the energy the food supplied, once you have removed the *cause* of emotional hunger it will not return.

Food will not remove the cause of emotional hunger so let's discuss ways in which we can.

CAUSES OF EMOTIONAL HUNGER

However the feelings that trigger emotional hunger show themselves, it basically comes down to feeling bad about yourself in some way: self-loathing, feelings of being useless, worthless, and unloved.

We are not only what we eat, we are also what we think. The mind and body are one unit, psychologically and physiologically connected. Therefore our thoughts can have a huge impact on our feelings and our health. The good news is that we can change physiological effects on our bodies by using our imagination and we can, without doubt, change our feelings and moods.

YOU ARE YOUR FIERCEST CRITIC

As a therapist I get to listen to what people say about themselves in private and it is astonishing how much self-abuse they put themselves through. They look in the mirror in the morning and say to themselves, 'I look old', 'ugly', 'my bum is huge', 'an elephant would be proud of those thighs', 'no wonder no-one likes me'. Is it any wonder they go through the day feeling so bad?

The point is that, while most people wouldn't take insults like that from others, they habitually and almost constantly insult themselves far more harshly than anyone else would.

TRY SOMETHING DIFFERENT

From now on treat yourself as kindly as you want others to treat you. If everyone insulted each other, as badly as we insult ourselves, we would all continually be beating each other up or worse. But we accept that kind of ill-treatment from ourselves, often with unpleasant and unhealthy psychological repercussions.

You will never motivate yourself to lose weight by being cruel to yourself or bullying yourself to meet impossibly high standards. You need to see self-loathing for what it really is and deal with it directly instead of trying to bury it under mountains of food.

Even as you begin the next phase – recognising you are a good, worthy, valuable individual – you may still experience some pangs of emotional hunger. At times when you feel down or have a low opinion of yourself look at the friends and family who can see the good, valuable and loveable traits in you.

What follows is a simple exercise to help you see what a wonderful person you really are and begin to be rid of those patterns of self-loathing.

Read through this exercise and understand what to do before practicing it.

Somebody loves you

1. Close your eyes and recall an image of a person – a family member, best friend or partner – someone who you know loves and appreciates you for who you are, not just for what you look like. Imagine that person is standing in front of you.

2. Move out of your body and step into the body of the person who loves you. See yourself through the eyes of that person. Feel the love and good feelings that person has for you. Really notice what it is that the person sees and appreciates in you. Notice and recognise the good qualities that person sees in you, qualities that perhaps you have not noticed in yourself.

3. Now go back into your own body and enjoy these good feelings knowing the good qualities that you are loved and appreciated for. Experience how good it feels to know you are loved and appreciated just as you are.

You can keep these good feelings all day long if you want, and you can repeat this exercise as often as you like to boost the effect. The more you do it the easier and more effective it becomes and you will automatically come to love and respect yourself all the time.

ANOREXIA, BULIMIA AND BODY DYSMORPHIA

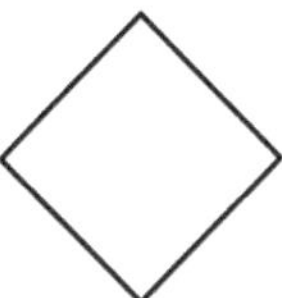

Hopefully this section will not apply to you in any way, but even so it is worth reading. It will provide an understanding of these conditions and the people who suffer from them. It will also ensure that through that understanding you will not become a victim.

Though the techniques in this book will make a real difference to the way you feel about yourself and the way you behave, they are not a substitute for professional help. If you know or suspect that you have an eating disorder you are advised to seek help from an appropriate professional.

People who suffer from anorexia or bulimia are often painfully thin, yet they are convinced that they are overweight. They never see how thin they really are, when they look in the mirror, they see a fat person. In most cases they don't even realise this.

Body dysmorphia prevents people from enjoying life or eating properly; at its worst, it can be fatal. Many sufferers focus on just a small part of themselves and direct all their self-loathing towards that aspect, some 'see' a totally distorted image of themselves in the mirror.

Sometimes sufferers hate themselves so much that they never notice the nice things others say about them. They never believe that anyone has said good or complimentary things about them. They are so totally convinced that there is nothing nice or good to be seen or said about them.

Our self-image mirrors what we think about ourselves so when we have a very poor self-image we automatically filter out any compliments that do not fit in with that poor image.

Once that poor self-image is replaced with self-love and self-respect your entire life changes for the better. You can enjoy life, enjoy and be proud of 'who' you are, with positive effect on everyone around you.

Everyone receives compliments and praise at some time in their lives and those positive, sincere compliments and words of encouragement that you receive, are an extremely valuable resource in helping you to appreciate your positive qualities and are very helpful in developing a good, positive self-image.

Using the following techniques before a mirror, will not only help to eliminate emotional hunger, but will also help you to feel better and more positive about yourself, and see the good person you really are when you look in the mirror.

As before, read through and understand the process before doing the exercises.

THE MIRROR OF LOVE – 1

1. Stand in front of a mirror with your eyes closed and remember a time when you received a compliment or praise from someone you respect or trust. You don't have to have believed it at the time but you must have trust in the sincerity of the person who said it. Go through the experience in your mind, making the memory as clear and strong as you can.

2. As you remember the praise or compliment, concentrate on the sincerity of the person who said it. Concentrate on your feelings of trust and respect for that person.

3. When you can feel that trust and regard for the person as strongly as possible, open your eyes. Look in the mirror and see what that person saw. Notice the good things that person saw in you and feel how good that feels.

4. Now imagine taking a photograph of yourself just as that person saw you. Take that photograph into your heart. Keep it safe there, and look at it any time you want to remind yourself of how good you can feel.

When you are practiced and comfortable with this part, go on to the next step.

THE MIRROR OF LOVE – 2

1. Spend at least one minute every day looking at yourself in the mirror, without clothes if this is comfortable for you, otherwise wear something that reveals your natural shape.

2. Notice what thoughts you get, they could range from 'why am I doing this?' to 'my arse is fat' to 'not too bad really'.

3. Whatever the thoughts, send love and approval and positive energy to the person in the mirror. Let that person know without doubt that you love that person regardless of size or shape.

Use these techniques every day. You will be pleasantly surprised at how soon you begin to notice changes, how quickly you move from self-hate to self-acceptance to self-love.

When you begin to meet your own emotional needs your emotional hunger will diminish. You will find yourself only eating when you are hungry and only eating enough to satisfy that hunger.

You will soon notice how much more confident you are and naturally start wearing clothes and doing things that you previously only dreamed of.

HOW IS YOUR BODY MEANT TO BE?

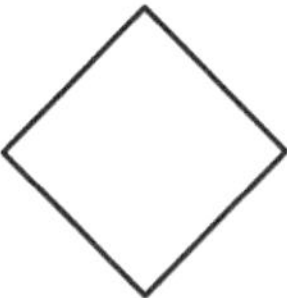

Very few women are naturally predisposed to have a 'model figure', in fact research suggests that thinness is actually a unique phenotype[6] which is also referred to as obesity resistance. Yet people who think of themselves as overweight spend half their lives comparing themselves with images in magazines of 'stick thin' models, making themselves feel bad about their own bodies. They then go away and eat too much in order to comfort themselves.

Most of these models are potentially highly stressed and anxious about their careers and appearance, leading them to constantly monitor everything which they eat and drink in order to maintain the body shape which is essential to their industry. Furthermore, most of the photos in magazines are airbrushed to hide any imperfections – in short they are artificial images and to a great extent not the 'real women' as they appear in everyday life.

The average person is designed to be around 5 or 6 feet tall (obviously there are exceptions to this due to inherited tendencies, genetics, and specific racial characteristics) and to have a natural shape that is the shape which our personal build, bone structure and race define for us, there is no ideal template which every person fits.

When we get too much fatter or thinner than that it is because we have messed things up by our actions. We get fat by consuming far more food than our bodies need, bodybuilders get

---

[6] Bulik, C M, and Allison, D B, 'The Genetic Epidemiology of Thinness', *Obesity Reviews*, vol. 2 (2001) p.107.

unnaturally over muscled through excessive exercise routines and eating abnormal amounts of protein. Also, in some cases, using chemicals means to 'cheat' nature and increase muscle bulk.

They achieve what they are aiming for but at what cost to their health and quality of life? How many stories do we hear about models or celebrities going into clinics to get treatment for addiction to drugs or alcohol?

So many people don't like their bodies, or their looks, sometimes to the extent of ignoring them – this is such a mistake – it is very important to pay attention to your body. If you want to change how it looks you must first learn to accept your natural body, the more you accept it as it is, the easier and more naturally it changes. You must make friends with the body you have, in order to get the body you want.

Even though you are working towards a slimmer waist, slimmer thighs, smaller bottom, or whatever it is you want. It will still be the body you are already in so you may as well get to love it now.

'*ANYONE INTERESTED IN THE GYM?*'

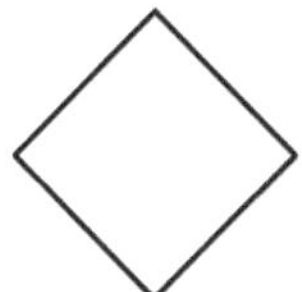

MYTHS OF METABOLISM

Metabolism is the chemical process within the body, which is essential for life. Some substances are broken down to yield energy whilst others are synthesised. The faster the metabolic rate, the faster everything happens, from changing body temperature to digesting food and converting it into energy. And, more to the point, the faster the metabolic rate, the faster it will burn off excess fat, whether the fat comes from the food we eat or from that stored in the stomach, hips and thighs.

The rate, or speed, of your present metabolism is called the 'base metabolic rate' and that primarily determines the amount of calories you burn each day. This does, of course, change with the amount of movement you perform each day.

A much-vaunted myth about metabolism put about in the diet and weight-loss business is 'some people have more difficulty than others in losing weight because their metabolism is slower' – RUBBISH!

Your metabolism changes all the time depending on how you use your body and how and what you eat: it is not fixed at any given rate.

What that means is that it is possible to control your own metabolic rate at will and, in this chapter, I will show you how to speed up and even supercharge your metabolic rate, increase the base rate and burn more calories each day, even when you are asleep.

You may well ask if simply changing your diet will alter your metabolism – the short answer is no. The simple truth is that if you continue to diet you will continue to regain weight.

As I explain more about metabolism you will soon see that the best thing to do with dieting is to stop doing it.

I have already said that if you starve yourself the body goes into fat-storing mode, storing as much fat as it can for future use in case the food supply runs out. To do this the metabolic rate will slow down to conserve energy.

However, if you eat whenever you are genuinely hungry the body gets to know that the energy it uses will always be replaced so there is no need to store fat. Your metabolism will consequently speed up to provide energy quickly and efficiently, helping you to stay thinner and have abundant energy for the more active person you will become as you get slimmer.

WHAT ABOUT THE GYM THEN?

If you really want to pound away on the treadmill or hump lumps of heavy metal around then go for it – but I'm guessing most people reading this volume would rather not. The good news is, there is no need to.

It is commonly thought that to increase metabolism you need to take lots of exercise. Now, before that sends you screaming for the door, I know the word exercise conjures up images of pounding endlessly on a treadmill or pumping iron in the gym. However, in truth, whatever you do that causes you to breathe more deeply and increases your heart rate more than normal (yes that is included) is exercise.

What can you think of that you would enjoy doing that would increase your heart rate and breathing? (Oh, come on. Is that all you can think about?). If you can think of something, you already know a way to supercharge your metabolism easily and enjoyably.

You already exercise every day just by getting out of bed and going about your daily business. All you need do to increase your metabolism and burn off more calories and excess weight is do a bit more of what you already do.

SUCCESS

Our bodies are designed to be used. We are equipped with muscles that are meant to be active just as our ancestors' were when they had to hunt for their food. Nowadays most of us have sedentary jobs. We use powered transport instead of our legs. Although we still have the genes for a fast-burning metabolism, we tend not to put them to their intended use.

A study by Dr James Hill revealed that on average a woman takes around 5,000 steps a day and a man takes around 6,000. Overweight people average 1,500 to 2,000 less than those who are the right weight.[7]

In terms of being slimmer that means you only need to take 2,000 extra steps a day to get to your ideal weight. The more steps you take the more you speed up the metabolism and burn off more calories plus the increased metabolism continues to burn more calories even when you are asleep. This is because as you take more steps your muscles become more toned and stronger; the more toned the muscles, the more they burn calories, even in sleep.

You only have to look at people who practice even moderate weight training to see that they rarely have any excess fat at all and that is because their toned muscles are burning calories even when they are asleep.

Though doctors recommend taking about 10,000 steps daily, even more remarkable and amazing weight-loss will be achieved by doubling that.

A cheap and simple pedometer, which can be obtained from most sports shops, will give you a pretty accurate count of how many steps you take in a day. Increasing this by around 2,000 steps a week will make a significant difference and as you become fitter you will easily be able to keep increasing the number of steps until you reach the target of between 10,000 to 20,000 steps daily.

You might say, 'But I haven't the time to walk that much', *RUBBISH*! All you need do is park the car a bit further from your destination; take the stairs instead of the lift; take a brisk stroll

---

[7] Hill, James O; Wyatt, Holly R, *Role of Physical Activity in Preventing and Treating Obesity*, Journal of Applied Physiology, 1999, pp.765–770

round the office during the break; a ten to thirty minute walk in the evening will do the trick. You will very soon see and feel the amazing difference.

Another thing you may notice about 'thin' people is that they are rarely, if ever, still. Even when they are sitting down relaxing they fidget – moving their hands, feet, legs, changing position, getting up to do things then sitting down again. All those little movements burn even more fat.

IT IS AS SIMPLE AS THAT

You have probably heard the phrase 'no pain, no gain' bandied about with reference to exercise. It is just not true, 'no effort, no gain' is much nearer to the truth. Just a small amount of effort will produce amazing results, and as you know, if you experience pain when taking exercise, you should stop. Exercising your body should be enjoyable and, of course, if you are enjoying it you will tend to do more, won't you?

Regular exercise has so many benefits you not only lose weight. You feel great, more lively and energetic because during exercise the body produces natural endorphins, a stress-reducing chemical in the brain.

When we are threatened or feel in danger the body goes into 'fight or flight' mode. It also does this when we are worried or wound up about something. As there is generally nothing to actually fight or run away from, this produces tension and stress, the lack of ability for the body to release this, can ultimately lead to illness.

Exercising helps the body to release those tensions, making us calmer and healthier with less likelihood of illness, or heart problems. Exercise triggers the natural process of rest, relaxation and recuperation; that pleasant, satisfying feeling that comes from vigorous movement. Exercise also causes us to feel great because of the release of endorphins which are the body's natural opiates.

Exercise improves your mood, making you feel happier, more able to cope and increases the ability to relax and sleep better.

Any time you are feeling a bit low, just go for a brisk walk, do the vacuuming, or exercise in some other way. Anything that increases your heart rate and breathing, you will soon find your mood lifting.

THERE'S AN ATHLETE IN YOU SOMEWHERE

Exercising helps build muscle, strengthen bones, lose fat, feel great, helps with clearer skin, improves mental alertness and increases sex drive, plus hormones released during exercise helps slow, or even reverse, the ageing process.[8]

WITH ALL THIS GOING FOR IT WHY AREN'T YOU DOING MORE?

One reason could well be because of the image you may have of sweat and pain in the gym, surrounded by people make you feel like going home and burying yourself under the duvet.

What you need to do is get rid of the negative associations with exercise and develop new, positive ones. Until then you will continue to tell yourself you should do it then get despondent because you don't.

The following technique will help you create an anchor, or trigger, that will help you feel great and increase your motivation, the trigger, or anchor, can be something simple and not too obvious that you can use any time you wish. It can be pressing the middle finger and thumb of one hand together making a fist, or stroking your earlobe – anything that you feel comfortable with.

As before, read through the steps and understand what you have to do before actually doing it.

GET MOTIVATED – 1

Shortly, I will ask you to recall a time when you felt really motivated or when you were doing something that you really enjoyed. Create an association with those good feelings and activating your trigger (squeezing your finger and thumb or whatever you chose). This will create a neural path in the brain, associating the trigger with the good feelings. The more you

---

[8] Miley, William, *The Psychology of Well Being*, Praeger Publishers: Westport (1999) p.17.

repeat it the stronger and more effective it gets so you need to do this over and over again.

1. Decide on a scale of 1 to 10 how strong your motivation to exercise is, 1 being very little, 10 being very strong.

2. Think of something that you are already strongly motivated to do – a hobby, being with loved ones, going to a favourite place. If nothing comes to mind, ask yourself how motivated would you be to accept a gift of a million pounds, rescue a loved one in danger, tell the boss to get stuffed if you won the lottery.

3. Whatever you choose to motivate you, visualise the scene clearly in your mind. Imagine it is actually happening, see and hear what you would see and hear. Experience the powerful emotions and feel just how being truly motivated feels. Notice every detail of the event, the sights, sounds, smells, colours make everything brighter, richer, stronger. Build up the feelings and sensations to a soaring peak and as you reach that peak, activate your chosen trigger.

4. Keep repeating that motivational scene in your mind, going over it again and again, each time feeling that powerful motivation and activating the trigger. Live it. Make it as real as possible, associating that trigger with the powerful motivational feelings all the time.

5. Now relax your trigger, step back and do something else for a minute…

6 Now let's test that trigger – activate your trigger, see how the motivational feelings come back. Remember, it may not be as powerful but those feelings will get stronger every time you repeat this exercise.

GET MOTIVATED – 2

Now we can make the association between feeling motivated and getting some exercise. Remember to read through this before practicing it.

1. Activate the trigger and get those feelings of being motivated, now imagine yourself doing some exercise, walking briskly, going through your day easily and actively. Imagine everything going exactly the way you want, finding more opportunities to move your body more than you normally would. See what you would see, hear what you would hear, feel the good feelings and exhilaration of moving your body. When you have done that, repeat it again, all the while keeping your trigger activated, permanently associating it with motivation to exercise.

2. Now test yourself on the scale of 1 to 10 to see how motivated you are to exercise, if you are in the high numbers you will easily be able to introduce more exercise and movement into your daily routine. If you are in the lower numbers you will need to practice these techniques a bit more, the more you practice the more powerful your motivation to exercise and succeed will become.

No matter how much you want to change it is important to remember that change can only happen one day at a time – if you were to drop a stone in weight overnight you would most likely die, and if you drop weight too quickly your skin will look like a deflated balloon. These things need to be done at a natural rate.

It is not strictly necessary to begin a formal exercise regime, though that would improve your appearance, and potentially enhance your moods and sex life, but you do need to use your body more. Increase the number of steps you take each day, dance, play sports, enjoy your life – enjoy the only body you have.

A FINAL WORD ABOUT EXERCISE

For women in particular, a simple exercise routine involving free weights (dumbbells etc.) is extremely beneficial. Exercising with free weights not only tones the muscles, but strengthens and increases the density of the bones. This is extremely good for the prevention of osteoporosis to which women can be susceptible.

There is no need to train to the extent that body builders do and there is no need to buy expensive weights. Empty plastic milk bottles filled with water or sand are perfectly adequate and the weight can easily be adjusted to suit by increasing the amount of water or sand is in each bottle.

Exercise routines can be found in all sorts of women's and men's, magazines or in books from the library.

CONTROLLING CRAVINGS

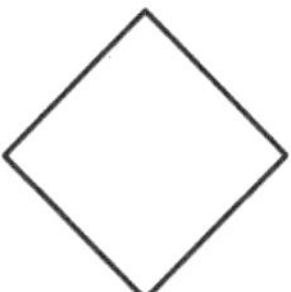

You may at times have cravings for a certain foods, chocolate, or cakes, and those cravings are urgent, needing to be satisfied immediately.

Those cravings are a learned behaviour and they can be un-learned.

You were not born with those cravings' you have developed and learned them for any number of reasons. The good news is they can be un-learned quite easily, sometimes in only a few minutes.

The first technique I am going to show you in a moment can reduce any food craving you may currently have in a couple of minutes. If you want to remove a specific food craving for ever then just go straight to the second technique.

REDUCING CRAVINGS TECHNIQUES: THE SLIM PERSON WITHIN YOU

Whenever you feel strong cravings for a particular food, simply follow this exercise and the craving will vanish as if by magic. This technique is based on the Meridian therapy called FREEWAY-CER ©, originated by Tom Bolton and Beverley Anderson. It is a very powerful tool for problems and issues of all kinds and is used here with their permission.

If you follow this technique exactly you can have complete control over your craving. You will need to concentrate and keep thinking of the food for which you have a craving.

Once more, read through the instructions carefully before beginning.

FREEWAY-CER ROUTINE©

1. Choose a focus word or short focus phrase to help you concentrate on the food you are craving. Measure the intensity of that craving on a scale of 0-10. Zero being no feeling at all and 10 being as powerful as it has ever felt.

2. Sit comfortably, eyes closed. Take 3 long slow deep breaths without straining then have a nice big luxurious *YAWN*. Repeat the focus word or phrase aloud once after each breathe and remember to keep breathing slowly and gently throughout the whole process.

3. Find the mid-brow point (just above the centre of the eyebrows in a small indent in the forehead) and with the tips of the index and middle fingers together, tap gently about 10 times then press this point and circle clockwise several times for about 10 seconds, breathing normally as you do.

4. Now make a loose fist with your left hand and place it in the centre of your chest just below the collar bone. Gently and lightly tap that central area about 10 times.

5. With the tips of the index and middle fingers of the right hand lightly tap the centre of the left palm 10 or more times then with the tips of the 4 fingers of the right hand tap the inner left wrist 10 or more times.

6. With the tips of the index and middle fingers of the left hand lightly tap the centre of the right palm 10 or more times then with the tips of the 4 fingers of the left hand tap the inner right wrist 10 or more times.

7. With the tips of the 4 fingers and the thumb of the left hand tap the centre of the bottom right rib (in line with the nipple) lightly 10 or more times.

8. With the tips of the 4 fingers and the thumb of the right hand tap the centre of the bottom left rib (in line with the nipple) lightly 10 or more times.

9. Now rescale the craving between 10 and 0. In the

unlikely event that the craving has not completely gone, simply go through the whole sequence again, focussing on the craving as before, but this time with lesser intensity.

10. When finally down to zero do the following: Put the palms of each hand over your ears and say aloud and convincingly three times: 'I have now let go of this (name the food) for ever. Put your hands comfortably back into your lap and have a nice big *YAWN*.

If you want to take it one stage further, and actively dislike the idea of eating that food, follow the next technique.

NO MORE CRAVINGS

The following technique is used to help clients who have a craving for a particular food, and never to want to eat that particular food again. It works in only a couple of minutes.

Most people turn to sugary foods to give themselves a 'treat' in order to lift their spirits. The problem is, all it usually does is add more weight to the stomach, hips and thighs.

Do not use the following unless you really do want to stop eating a particular food for ever. If you only want to control your cravings, stick to the previous 'reducing cravings' method.

Read through the technique carefully before proceeding.

1. Think of a food you absolutely hate, one you find completely revolting. If there isn't one, think about a plate of worms, maggots, dead rats.

2. Now, imagine there is a large plate of that food you hate in front of you, vividly imagine it as though it is really there. Imagine looking at it, smelling it and then eating it, all the while squeezing one hand into a fist. Really, vividly imagine eating that food, how it feels in your mouth. Still squeezing your fist, imagine how it tastes, how it feels sliding down your throat, until you feel completely revolted. When you get to feeling like you might throw up, stop and relax your hand.

3. Now think of the food you want to stop eating, chocolate or whatever, while you think of it, imagine what a plate of it looks like.

4. Now make that image bigger, brighter. Make the plate of food huge until it is bigger than you. Even bigger than that, make it bigger and bigger, getting closer and closer to it until you pass right through it and come out the other side.

5. Squeeze your fist so you recall the taste of the food you find revolting while imagining eating some of the food you like. Now imagine eating the food you like together with the revolting food. Imagine eating both foods together, the one you love and the one you hate, keep imagining this in your mind, a massive plate of it, swallowing it down, all the while keeping, the fist clenched. Go on, eat more and more until you are ready to burst or vomit then stop.

6. Now think about the food you used to like and notice how you are no longer interested in it.

Repeat this exercise as often as you need until the craving is completely eliminated.

SOME FINAL WORDS OF ENCOURAGEMENT

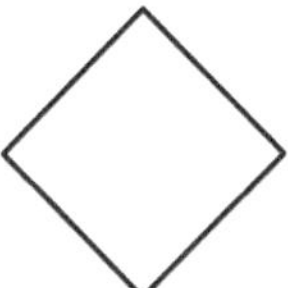

The Healthy Mind, Beautiful Body weight-loss system really is as simple as it sounds. Furthermore, it really does work.

Even if you are grossly overweight right now this system will work for you. There is no need to go on any kind of diet before using this system. In fact, my advice is do not go on any diet ever – they do not work permanently and will ultimately make you fatter.

As with anything new you will probably make mistakes or forget to follow the system for a while. You may even slip into the odd binge eating session, please do not let it bother you, just get back on the bike and start again, it pays to be relaxed and easy about this. No food police are going to come round and bash your head in for the odd slip-up. This system is designed so that you can enjoy eating.

Because of brainwashing from the diet industry some people may feel guilty for eating the food they like rather than what they're told they should. As long as you only eat when you are hungry and stop as soon as you are full, unless your diet consists entirely of junk food, just eat what you like. Follow the Four Basic Principles in this book and everything will fall into place – and your excess fat will fall off.

Some may find it difficult to break out of the 'eat everything on the plate' habit because of ingrained programming as a child, for instance. If this is the case, try removing some food from the plate before eating then eat what is left, or serving yourself a smaller portion to begin with. If you are still hungry you can always take more afterwards. Also, don't rely on willpower alone;

use your imagination as explained in this book. Your imagination is far more powerful than willpower.

If you really will not or cannot do any extra exercise, you will still lose weight with this system. However, by being just a bit more active than you usually are, you will lose weight even more quickly – so why choose the slow route? It's not a good idea to go at the whole thing furiously, trying to lose weight immediately. Take it one step at a time. Increase activity gradually each week and you'll feel in control and will be able to keep it up for life. Remember, it is not safe to lose more than 3 or 4 pounds a week. If you were to drop a stone overnight you would probably get very ill or even die. To be sure of how much weight is safe for you to lose each week see your GP.

However, please do not keep weighing yourself, scales are not that helpful. If you keep weighing yourself without giving this system time to work you will only set yourself up for failure. It is far better to be aware of how much better you are getting. Humans don't stand still – we are either getting better or getting worse. If you're getting better then great, keep it up; if you're getting worse, then you know which way you need to go.

Finally, remember it isn't the system itself that works; it's you using the system that works.

Just follow the Four Basic Principles:

1.   Eat when you're hungry.

2.   Eat the foods you like, not what you think you ought.

3.   Eat slowly, chew thoroughly and enjoy every mouthful.

4.   Stop the moment you think you are full.

YOU CANNOT FAIL UNLESS YOU STOP TRYING

So please continue to read and practice all the exercises in this book regularly, particularly the Freeway routine. Keep listening to and using the CD, at least every other day, until you feel the changes occurring within you. If you find yourself faltering later, then go back to it and use the motivation to drive yourself forward.

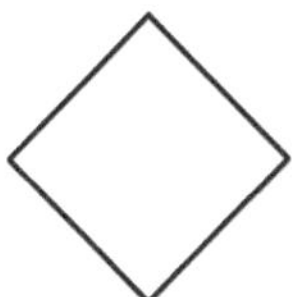

WITH THE HEALTHY MIND BEAUTIFUL
BODY REVOLUTIONARY WEIGHT RELEASE
SYSTEM YOU CAN:

EAT THE FOODS YOU LIKE, WHENEVER
YOU LIKE, AND STILL LOSE WEIGHT.

BECOME REALLY HAPPY WITH YOUR
BODY.

EASILY RESIST EXCESS FOOD AND
CRAVINGS.

LOSE WEIGHT WITHOUT EXERCISING.

I WANT TO HEAR ABOUT YOUR SUCCESS

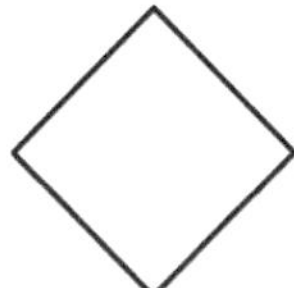

You can e-mail me at *berniemorganmindtherapist@gmail.com;*

Visit my website at *www.berniemorgan.com;*

Visit the FREEWAY-CER website at *www.freeway-cer.com,*

Or you can write to me c/o Clear Mind Therapy, The Orchard, Clevedon Lane, Clapton in Gordano, North Somerset, BS20 7RH.

You can also use these contact details if you are interested in having one-to-one therapy sessions or would like to organise a group seminar in your area.

If you have any problems with any aspect of this book and the Healthy Mind, Beautiful Body system, please contact me. I will do my best to help.

My thanks and best wishes to you.

9 781844 018185